RESISTANCE LOOP BAND MANUAL

TOTAL BODY HOME EXERCISE WORKBOOK FOR FAT LOSS AND STRENGTH

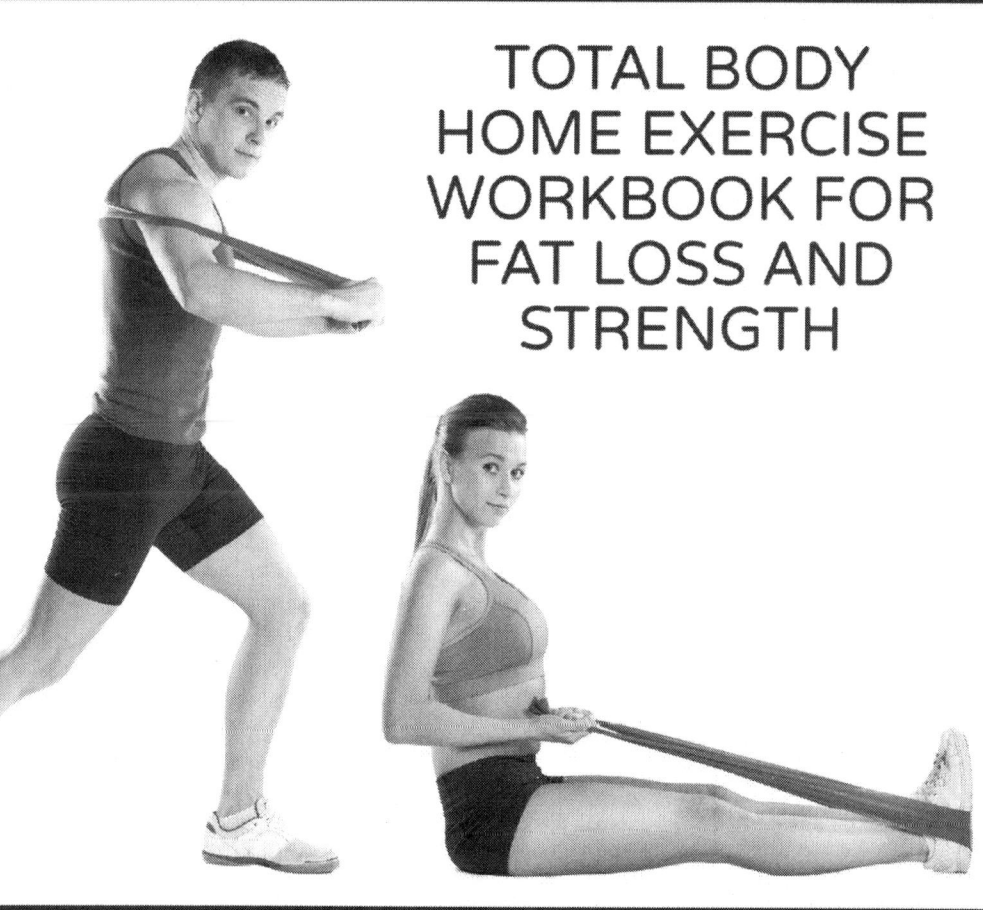

ALICIA LABERT

Introduction

If you are reading these words, then I believe an inner urge has developed within you to make yourself fit, have a great body and lead a healthy lifestyle. But that doesn't come cheap; the dream is definitely more expensive than the equipment you purchased for this purpose. The currency to attain this dream of yours is dedication, hard work and sweat. I say these words as an experienced follower of resistance training. Lots of people start with a good intention but lose out their steam owing to slow and discouraging results, but with right knowledge and dedicated workout programs, it is simply a matter of time before you have a beautiful and a fit body.

Before going into this form of exercise and their benefits, let us get familiar with the fundamental laws of exercise. Since the resistance loop band use the resistance method of training, let's get to know it first.

Medical Disclaimer:

You should consult your physician before starting any exercise routine.

If you have any questions about any medical matter you should consult a doctor.

If during your workout you suffer from any medical condition you should seek immediate medical attention.

The recommendations in this document are for educational purpose only. The exercises contained in this book are for healthy individuals 18 years or older.

Before starting your exercise routine you should make sure that your resistance bands are in perfect condition. Always warm-up before your exercise. It is recommended to use yoga mat to perform exercises with resistance loop bands.

If you experience dizziness or shortness of breath you should stop exercising and consult your physician.

Chapter 1: What is Resistance training?

Resistance training is a form of exercise that forces the muscle to shrink in size owing to external stress with a goal that the impending results lead to increase in muscular size, mass, strength and toning of the targeted muscle.

Resistance training is a lot similar to weight training; in fact it is developed from weight training by adding the techniques that the modern technology has made possible. It is equally effective for both sexes, although the results may slightly vary due to difference in hormonal balance.

The principle that involves manipulating the body to attain the required result is a complex task but an attempt has been made to simplify it so that a person who has no outright knowledge in exercises can understand and start working out to improve their health.

Before starting any workout program, the first rule is to have clarity in your goal. It is whether you want to reduce your weight, burn the excess fat or build a particular muscle and increase your strength. Resistance training is a training method wherein lots of results are possible with little manipulation. Aerobic exercises can be used to reduce weight and fat, while lifting weights can increase muscle and strength. It is all a matter of making up your mind and setting your priorities.

The whole training process is divided into three segments

1. Work out
2. Food consumed
3. Sleep cycle

Workout is the exercise that you perform with an intention of reducing weight or increasing the muscular size. When you perform the actual exercise, the muscles contract and expand in a particular motion thus causing tears on a microscopic level. These tears are what make the muscle grow.

The food that you intake is an important part in making your body grow. The food consumed contains different substances such as protein and fiber that help the muscle to repair the microscopic tear which in turn increases the size of the muscle. When healthy food is not consumed, the nutrients required to rebuild the muscle is unavailable to the body and it shrinks back into its original form, thus making waste of the workout and causing fatigue.

The sleep cycle is as important as the workout and the food intake. Adequate sleep is very important for the body to repair itself. The actual process of repair takes place when your muscles are stationary and undisturbed state, i.e. when you are asleep. The recommended sleep period for a healthy lifestyle is 8 hours. But for people working out, the more you sleep, the healthier you become.

Weight reduction process takes place in a slightly different way, if your goal is to reduce weight and burn your fat, the following words will make a huge impact in your process to become healthy.

Fat is nothing else but energy that is stored in hibernated form. The body stores energy because it doesn't like to waste the energy that you have consumed. It stores it in a form of fat to utilize this energy when you don't supply food to the body.

To simplify the process, consider that when you eat food, you simply give your body energy to perform its daily physical activities such as walking, moving the limbs and other involuntary activities. Consider that the food you eat has 1000 units of energy, but your body needs only 800 units of energy. In this case, the body doesn't discard the energy, but simply converts it into fat and stores it in various parts of the body (your love handles around the waist has huge amount of energy).

To reduce the fat, the simple trick is to increase your physical activity such as walking, jogging, running, sprinting, cycling, jumping and exercising. When you increase the physical activity (aerobic exercises), your body consumes all the available energy, but if it requires more energy, it will simply take some of the fat from your body and reconvert it into energy and spend it on that physical activity.

Thus the goal is to consume less calories of energy and spend more by performing physical activity.

Consider that you need 500 units of energy when you perform an aerobic exercise, and your daily activities need 800 units of energy, that's a total of 1300 units of energy. But you only consume food giving 1000 units of energy. You burn 300 unit of extra energy by converting fat.

But if you reduce the amount of energy that you intake to 800 units, a total of 500 units of energy would be required by your body that will be taken by reducing the fat. For an average person with a medium sized pot belly, 6 month would be sufficient time to get into his fittest form.

Chapter 2: Resistance Loop Bands

What is a resistance loop band and how does it help you get into your fittest self?

Resistance loop bands are a modified version of the resistance tubes. The aim of this loop bands is to perform exercises and target the muscles that aren't possible with resistance tubes.

Since one size doesn't fit everyone, there are usually 4 different variations of the resistance loop bands.

1. Light weight
2. Medium weight
3. Heavy weight
4. Extra heavy weight

The band length will also vary according to the use.

The difference between the bands is elasticity. This is really important for a person working out based on his difficulty level, type of exercise being performed and the muscle targeted. The standing out feature of the resistance bands is their portability. They can be carried in your backpack or even in your pocket. **This simple piece of equipment allows you to perform wide range of exercises that can target almost any muscle without lowering the impact level much when compared to the traditional gym exercises targeting the same muscle**. It's like carrying a portable gym.

One of the benefits that you get using the loop band is that, when using the traditional weight, the amount of effort you put is constant. With this resistance loop band, as you stretch its limit, the resistance level increases in turn increasing the effort put up by the muscle. This variation in effort puts the muscle into a different kind of stress increasing its growth chances.

Chapter 3: Benefits of resistance loop band

Resistance loop bands offer wide range of benefits, some of them are mentioned below.

1) It's not only effective but also cost effective.

Nobody wants to spend their entire income on different kinds of gym equipment; these resistance loop bands offer same kind of results with virtually no cost at all. A resistance loop bands set usually varies in cost from $10 to $30 depending upon the elasticity weight level, size and length.

2) Adapts to different parameters

Everyone has to start from the scratch when it comes to fitness, hence you become a beginner. But as you go and adapt to the muscular movements, your body needs something more challenging to grow the muscles out of the shell. As bands come in different difficulty level, start with the light weight one and increase your difficulty level as you go with medium, heavy and extra heavy bands that challenge you to the extreme.

3) Variations in exercising.

Since the band can be used to stretch muscle in different motion, a variety of exercise types are possible with the resistance loop bands. As different types of exercises are required to expand a muscle to avoid muscle adaptability, these loop bands help in performing them without addition equipment. A great feature of resistance bands is that they can be used with other equipment to enhance your work out. For example attaching a weight and suspending from it your neck increases your net weight during a chin up or squat thus exerting more pressure on the targeted muscle.

4) Inventing your own exercise.

A cool feature with the resistance loop bands is that they allow inventing your own exercises thus encouraging the user to workout in an innovative and imaginative way.

5) Portability taken to the highest level.

As said earlier, the loop band fits just right into your pocket and will offer the same exercise methods which require traditional gym equipment without compromising on the impact level. It will be most useful to people who are busy with their jobs. They can perform the exercise whenever they get some free time and this type of exercise doesn't require much space. It can also be used by travelers who cannot stay at a place and find a gym nearby.

6) Workout without a gym partner.

A bench press with 80lbs on each side tends to call for a gym partner in case of unseen events. This resistance loop bands can be performed by a single person without any external help.

Chapter 4: Warm - up

Warm up before an exercise is severely under rated. It is one activity that will prevent your body from injuring the muscle while performing rigorous exercises. The sole aim of the warm up routine is to slowly raise the core temperature of the body and loosen up the muscle, preparing them for the upcoming strenuous activities.

In case the warm up exercises aren't performed, the muscles and the cardiovascular system which have been dormant for a while will undergo a lot of stress during the exercise, severely damaging itself. The warm up exercises puts low level pressure upon the various systems in the body and since they adapt quickly, the system will be ready for the following exercise routine which puts a bit more strain upon them.

The common type of warm ups exercises are

1. Jogging
2. Cycling
3. Skipping
4. Stretching of various muscles.

The aim of the warm up is just to prepare the body for the upcoming workout. It is to be kept in mind that not too much energy should be spent in the warm-up session as it leads to fatigue during the actual workout.

Some of the other specific warm-up exercises are.

Burpees.

Burpees are a whole body warm up exercise. To perform this exercise, simple stand on your legs firmly, bend down and touch the ground with your palms. Move your legs further and try to touch the ground using your waist stretching it completely. Then get back into the standing position. Perform this exercise for about 20 times.

Jumping jacks.

This exercise will warm up a lot of muscles and the cardio vascular system. First stand firmly, jump in the air while raising your hands laterally above your head and stretching your legs and landing on them firmly. Jump again and get back into the initial position.

Stretching

Stretching is an exercise which works with an aim to warm up specific muscles. Various exercises are available to target different muscle.

Inner Thigh Stretches

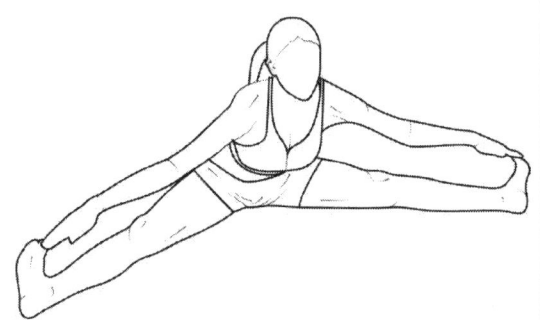

Side Bends

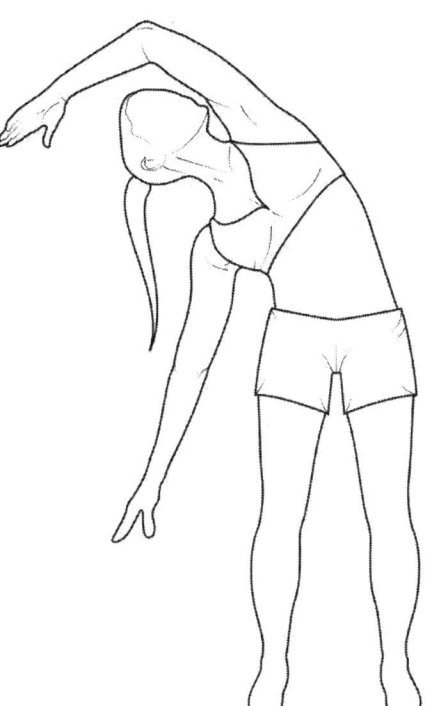

Forward Bend

Calf

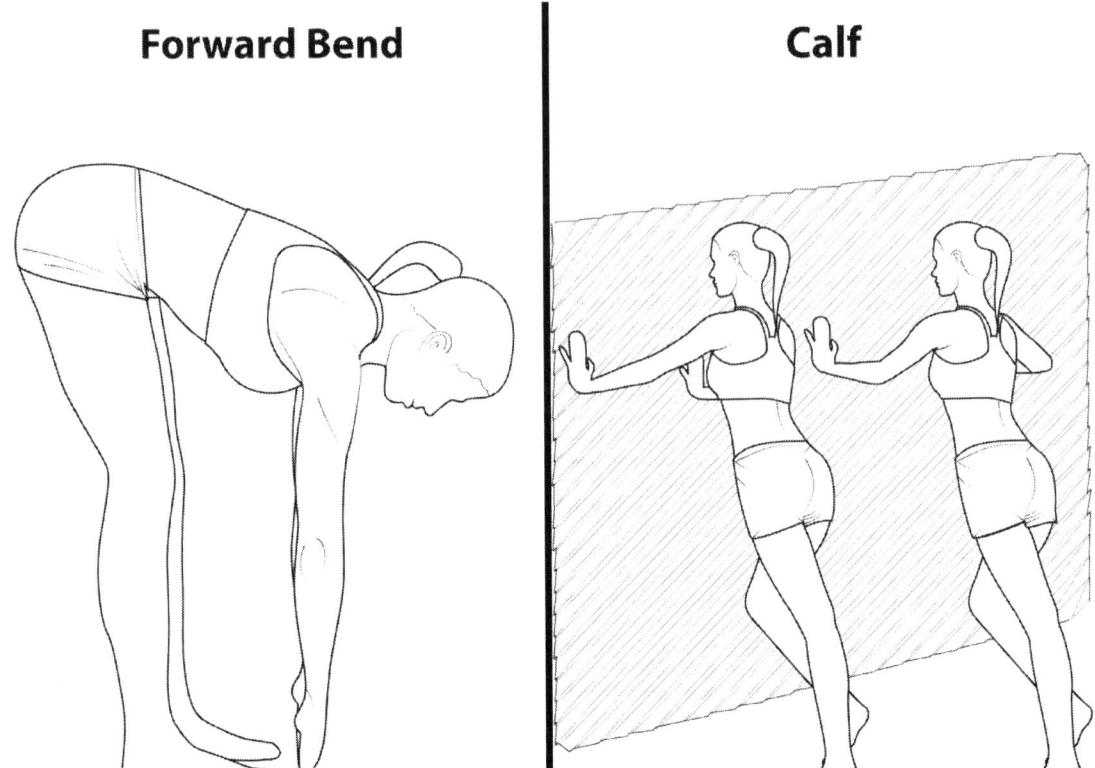

Chapter 5: Work out exercises

There are hundreds of muscle in your body and thousands of exercise to train them. Some of the exercise are described below to help you get a picture of how the loop band works and how does it affect your body.

<u>Upper body</u>

Lateral push up band walk. (Advance level)

This is an exercise that should only be performed by experienced people. Beginners performing this exercise will subject their muscles to strain they cannot take.

To perform this exercise, put your hands in the resistance loop band and suspend it against your forearm. The more the band is towards the wrist, the harder the exercise becomes. Now with the band suspended against your forearm, get into the push up position with the back, butt and legs forming a straight inclined line supported by your hands. Perform a push up and then move your right hand for about 5 inches to the right and then do the same with the left hand. It should be as it you are walking with your hands. Then move back to the initial position and perform a push up. Do it for 10 times for 2 sets.

Lateral Push Up Band Walk   Lateral Push Up Band Walk

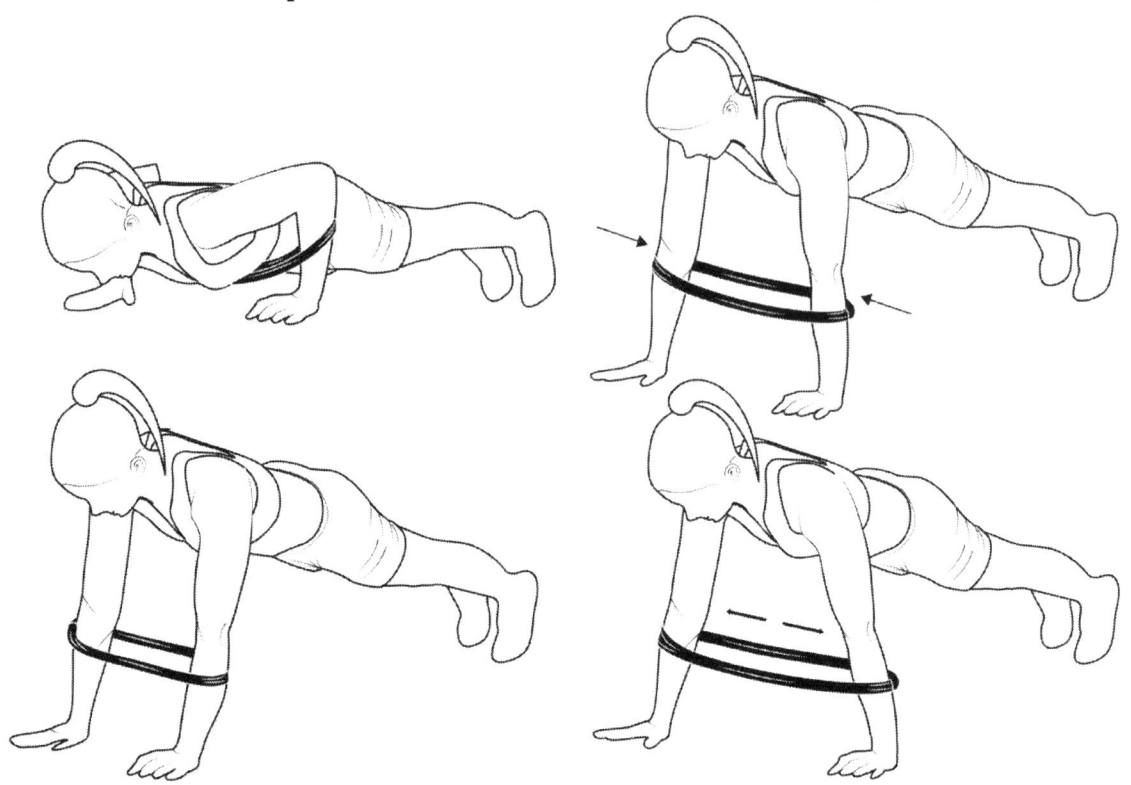

Cross chest triceps pushdown. (Beginner)

One of the few exercises that is precise in training the muscle and give you quick results is the cross chest triceps pushdown. To perform this exercise, stand straight with sufficient distance between the legs for stability. Take the resistance loop band and suspend it against your thumb and fore finger of your left hand while the rest of the band hangs freely. Grip firmly your right shoulder or the right side of your chest. Grip the remaining band with your right hand and pull it down in a straight line along your torso. Repeat for 8 to 12 times. Do it alternatively with the right hand for 3 sets.

Cross Chest Triceps Pushdown

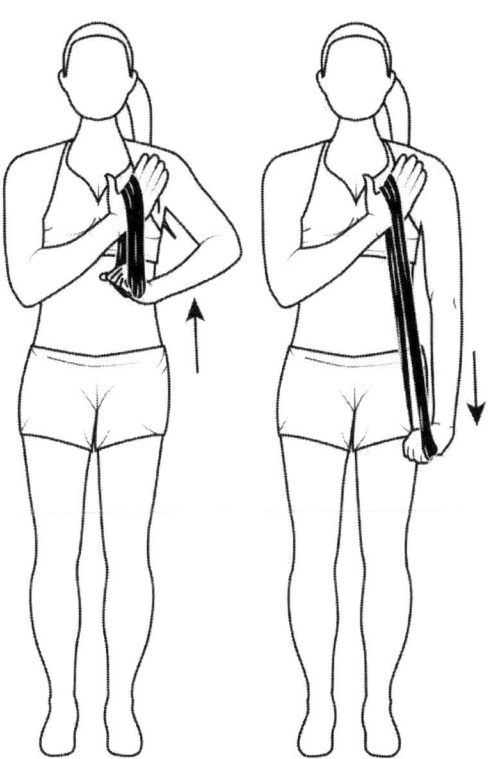

Lateral arm raise. (Beginner)

To perform this exercise, stand straight on the floor. You can also perform this exercise in a sitting position but the standing position is preferred for the comfortable movement of the muscles. Suspend the band around your hands at the forearm region. The closer the band is to the wrist, the harder the exercise becomes. The arm should be at the level of the chest. Pull the band so that the arms stretch beyond the shoulder distance and stay in the position for 5 seconds. Bring the hands to the initial position and repeat the process for 10 to 15 times.

Lateral Arm Raise

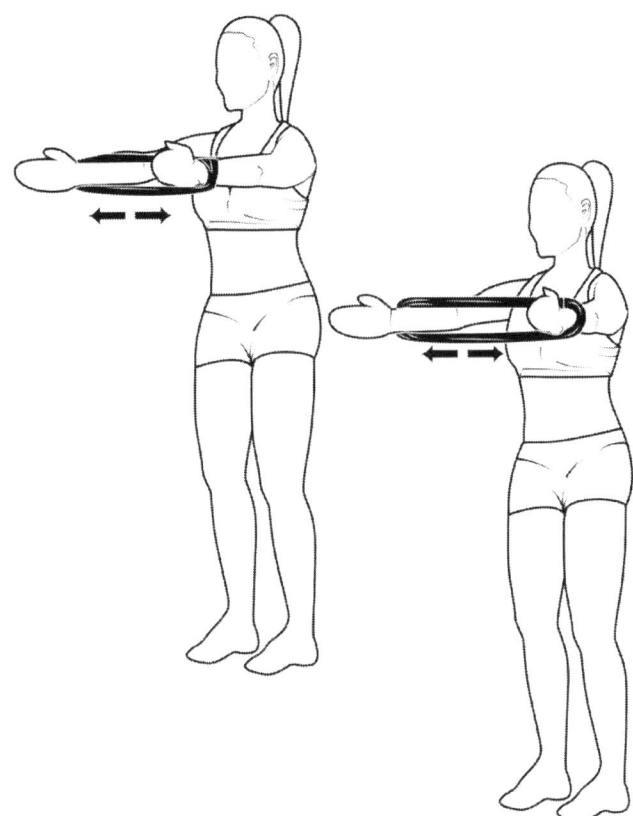

Bicep curl. (Beginner)

Bicep curl is an effective way to train your biceps using this resistance loop band. Every male wants a big and muscular arm and female, beautiful, slender and shapely arms that complement her figure. To perform this exercise get into a position one of your knee touches the ground while the other leg rests on the foot. Suspend the resistance loop band around your knee and pull the band to your shoulder level with the arm. Keep in mind that only the forearm and wrists should make the movement while the rest remains stationary. Repeat this to 15 times in 3 sets.

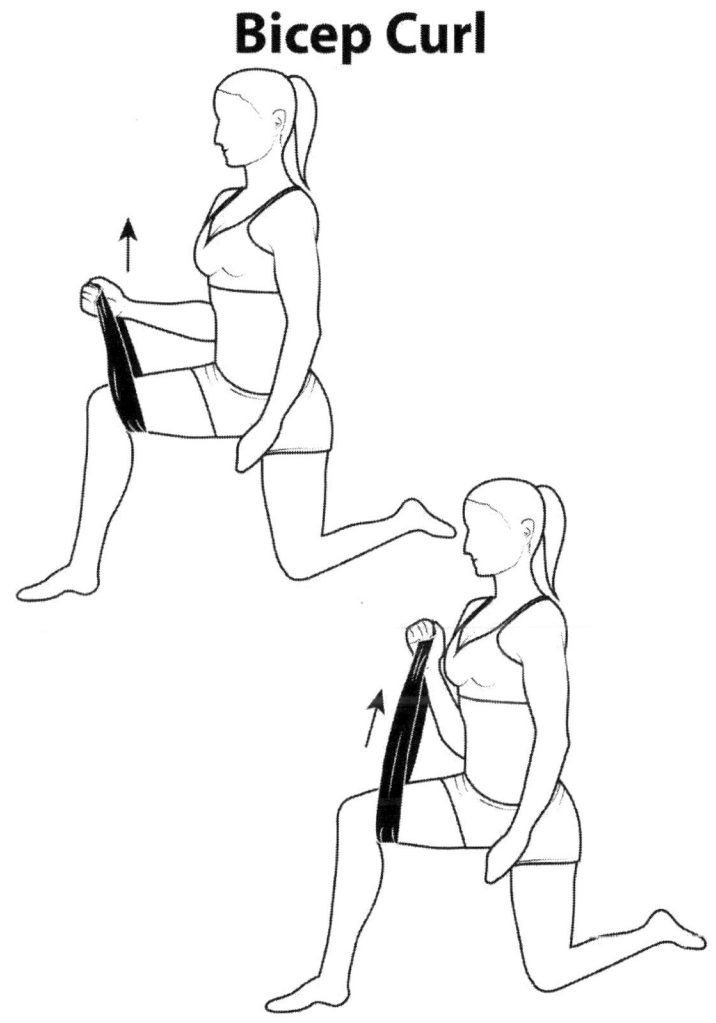

Behind the back extension. (Advance level)

This complex exercise shouldn't be performed by beginners. You can gradually pick up other form of exercises and gain some experience with the resistance loop band before trying out this exercise. To perform it, suspend the band around both of your forearm. Hands should levitate about 5 inches from your butt muscles. Now pull the band as far as you can with your arms. It is very important that the loop band doesn't touch the back or the butt muscles. Repeat it for 15 times to train your deltoids and region below the shoulder blades.

Behind The Back Extension

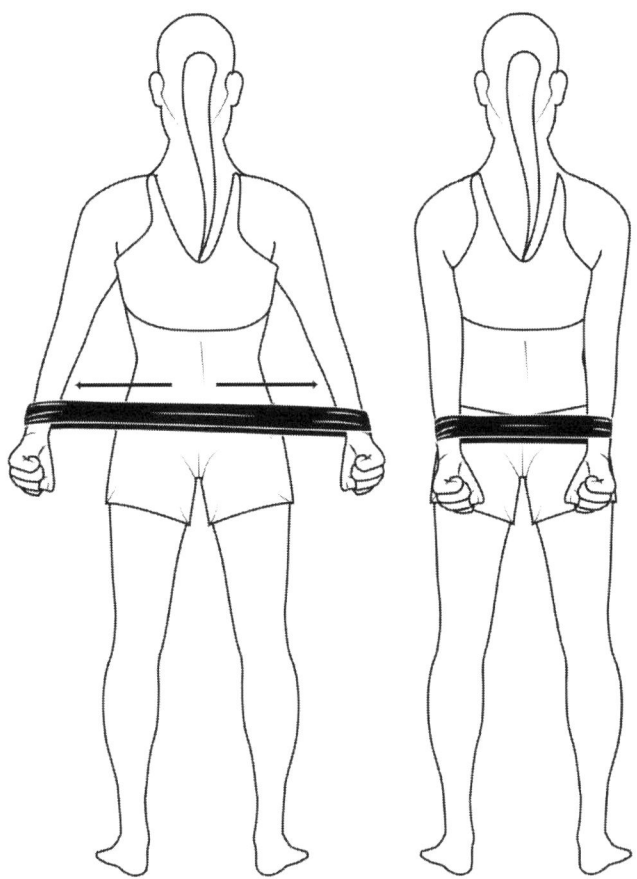

Vertical arm raise. (Beginner)

Vertical arm raises is a different type of exercise that targets the traps and the shoulder in a very effective way. To perform this exercise, stretch your hand in front of your chest in a vertical position. Suspend the resistance loop band around the hands. Pull apart the band in a vertical position until one hand is above your head and the other on your waist level. Repeat the same for about 8 to 12 times in 3 sets.

Vertical Arm Raise

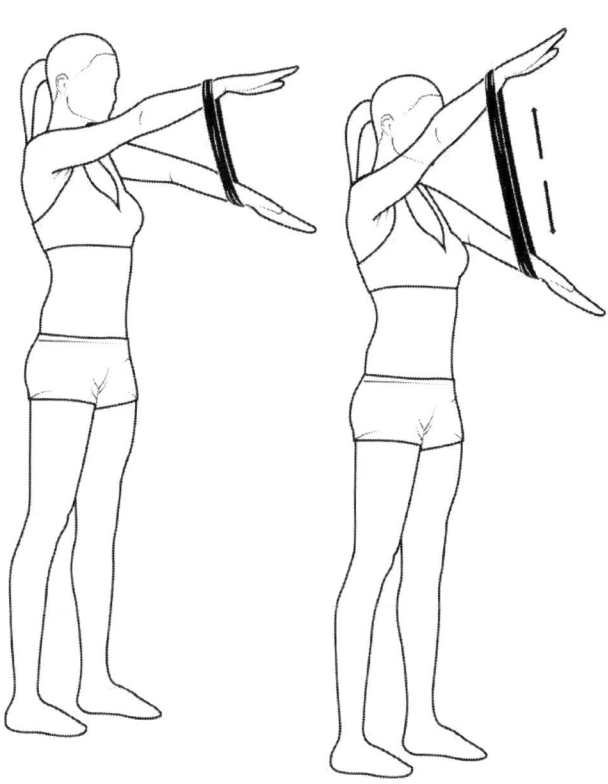

Side bends (Beginner)

To perform this exercise, stand firmly with your feet apart. The distance should be of shoulder length. Raise your hands over the head with the resistance loop band in your hands stretching it. Now slowly, by taking the air in, bend side wards simultaneously pulling the loop band apart. The back should be erect and the legs stationary. This exercise helps you to train your side stomach while reducing the fat in the waist region. Repeat for 20 times on each side.

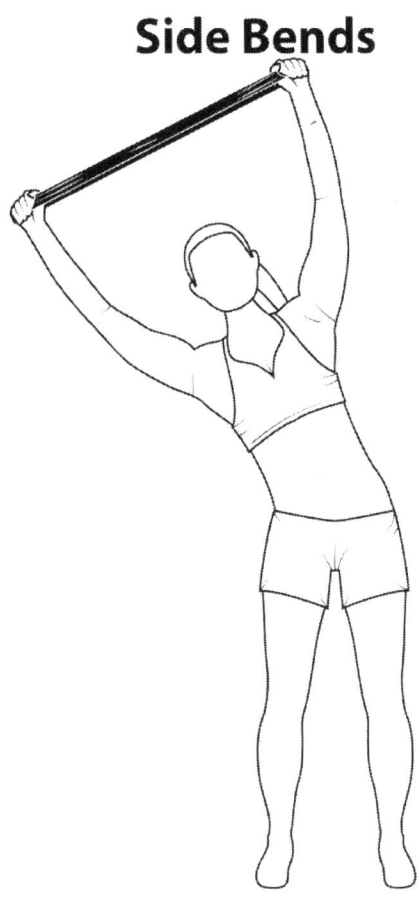

Single arm rowing (Beginner)

To perform this exercise, kneel down as if you are tying a shoe lace. Pin the resistance loop band under your left foot. Keeping your back a little inclined, pull the band to the extent that your wrist touches just below the arm pit. Perform this exercise for as long as you feel like doing and repeat the same for the left arm. This exercise targets lower back.

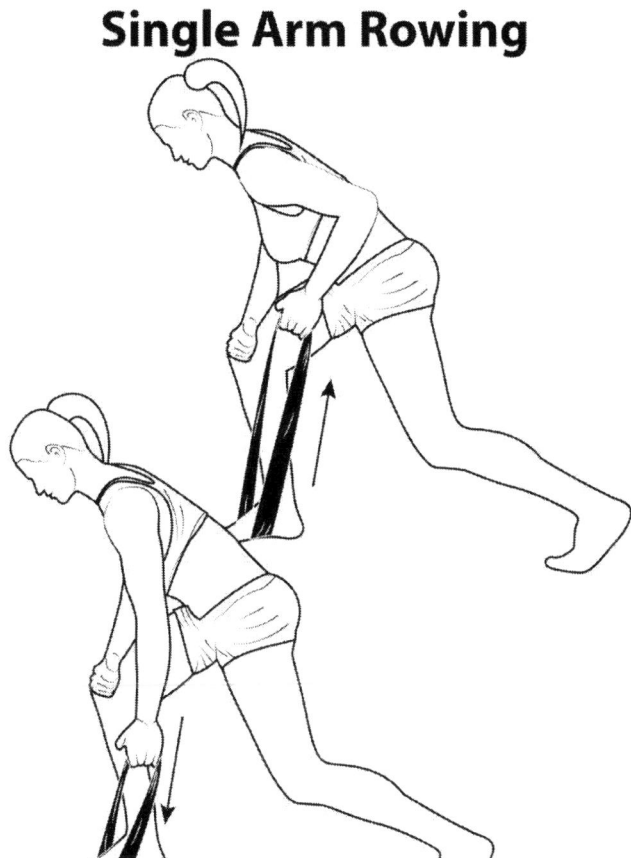

Triceps extension. (Beginner)

Triceps is one of the most ignored muscles of the body, but it has to be trained with dedication for the arm to look full in a male and curvy and slender in a female. To perform triceps extension, stand straight with your legs wide apart so that you have a firm grip on the ground. Take the resistance loop band in the arm that you want to train and slowly bring it down your back. Take hold of the other end with your free hand at your lower back region. Now the only motion should be of the hand that is to be trained. By keeping the hand at the lower back stationary, pull the resistance loop band in a straight motion above your head to the top till you can stretch. Repeat this exercise 8 to 10 times for 3 sets.
Train the other hand alternatively.

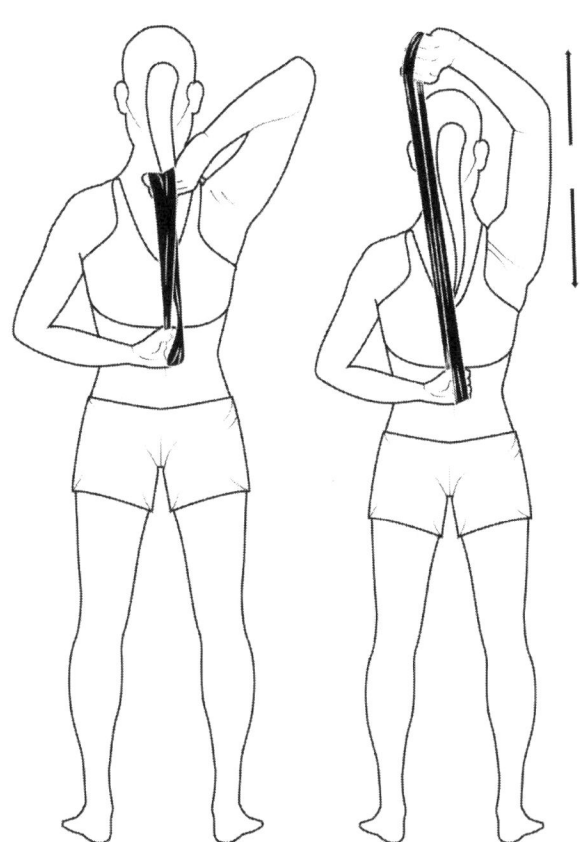

Triceps Extension

Bent arm front raises. (Beginner)

To perform this exercise, suspend the resistance loop band against your wrists, pull the band slightly so that a pressure is applied on the wrists. Now with your back against the wall and elbows touching the wall, raise both of the hands above your head level. The hands should be at a 45 degree angle at the elbow and should work in sync with each other. Repeat this exercise for 25 times.

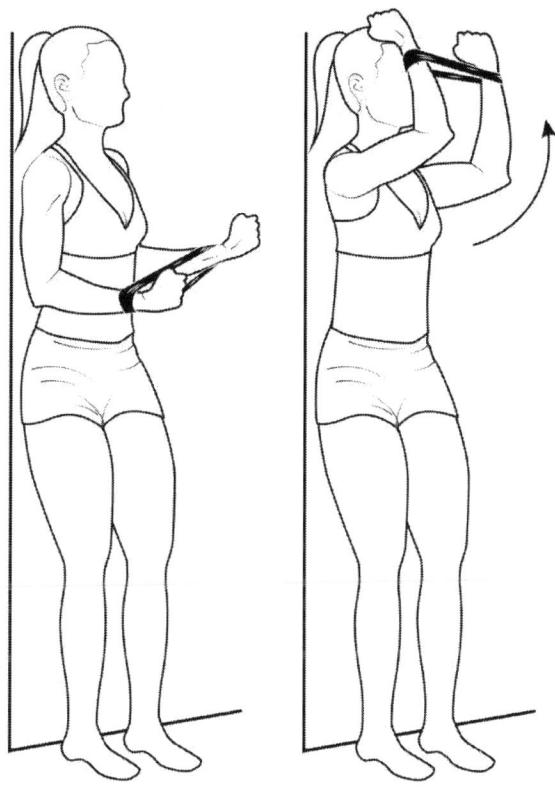

Resistive boxing. (Advance level)

This exercise is a dynamite of a workout bringing flexibility to the whole body. To perform this exercise, stand firmly on your feet with 2 feet gap between them. Grip the resistance loop band using your wrists. Consider an imaginary person in front and try to punch him on his left breast using the right hand and on his right breast using the left hand. All the while stretching the band and performing a semi squat motion.

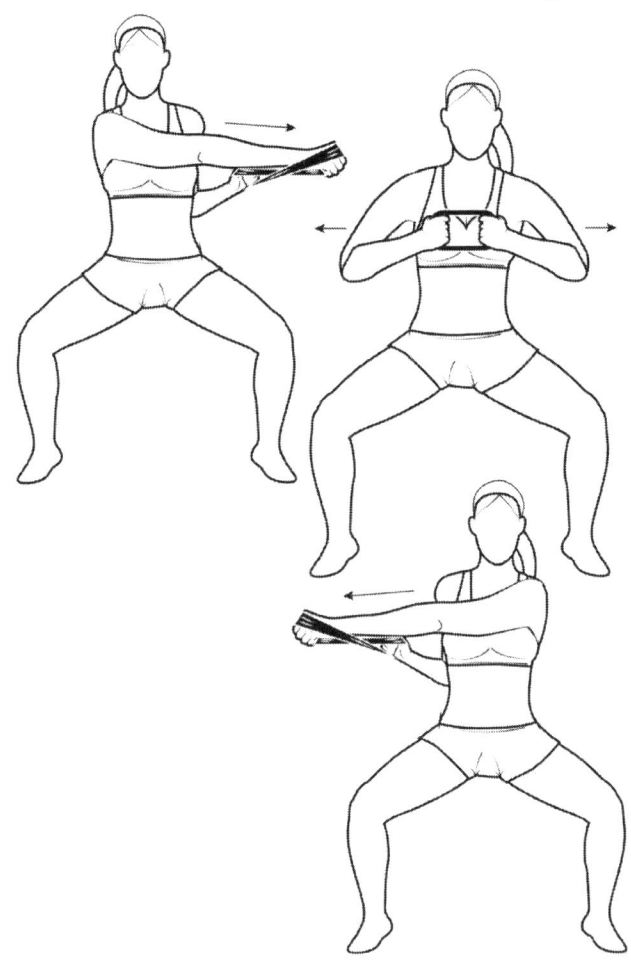

Shoulder rotation (Advance level)

This is an effective exercise to train your shoulders with the resistance loop band. To perform this exercise, stand firmly with your back touching the wall for support. Suspend the band against your wrists with the elbow touching the wall. Gently squeeze your wrists to their respective sides so that the right shoulder rotates right and the left one towards the left. Squeeze in and out to train your cuffs and shoulders. Repeat the process for about 25 times. This exercise has to be done slowly and increase the number gradually after multiple workout sessions.

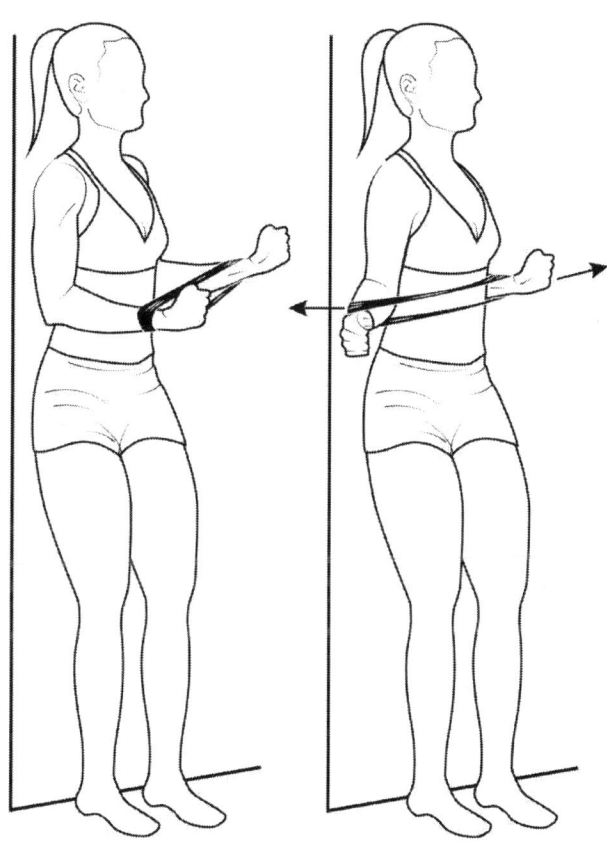

Lower body

Knee lifts (Beginner)

Wearing shoes is a must for this exercise. Place the resistance loop band on the toes of your shoes. The distance between the shoes should be 6 to 8 inches. Not more than that. Now stand in a firm position with your back straight and abs tightened. Lift your right foot to bring it to the position of the left knee. All the while the left leg should pin down the band so as to not lose the grip. Stay in this position for 5 to 7 sec. return to the normal position and repeat the same with the other leg. Do this 20 times.

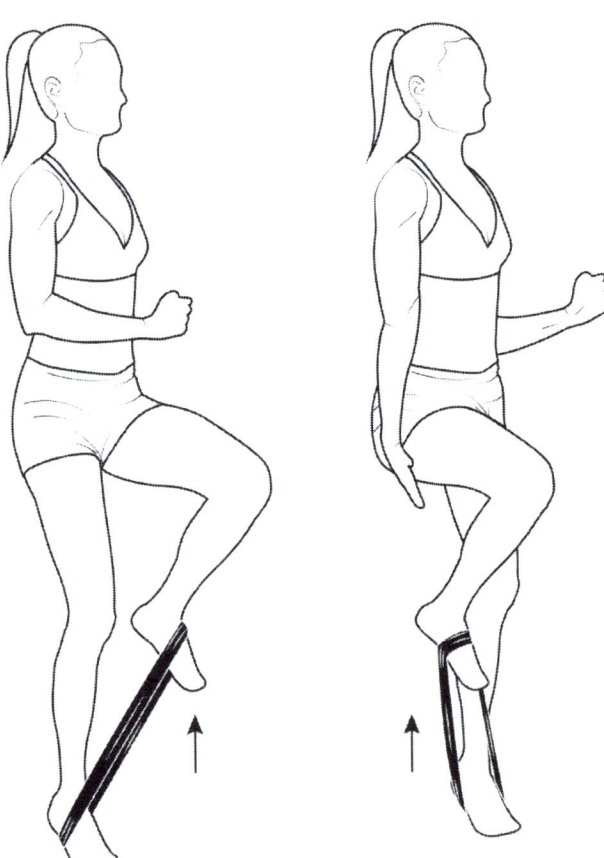

Kickbacks. (Beginner)

Place the resistance loop band around the area of your ankle such that they do not drop to the ground. Lie against the floor on your stomach. The entire weight of your legs should be on your toes. Tightening your butt muscles and the abs, raise your right leg towards the sky. Your back should be straight all the time and you should face the wall in front. Raise the leg as far as possible and bring it back to the initial position after a couple of minutes. Now raise the other leg to complete a repetition. Do this for 15 times and 3 to 5 sets. The stationary leg should rest on its toes.

Kickbacks

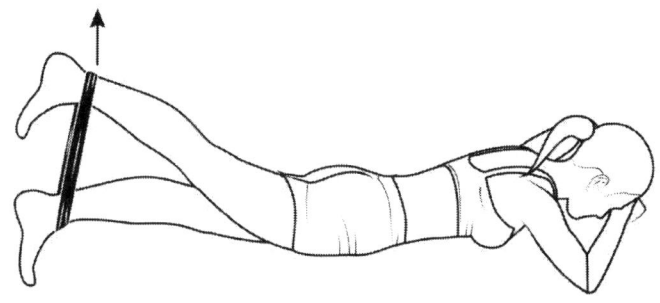

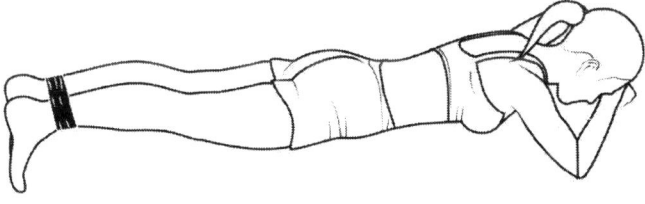

Clamshell. (Advance level)

This exercise is great for your gluteal muscles (butt muscles). Performing this exercise along with squats will develop a perfect butt that will complement your body in a great way. To perform this exercise, lie down comfortably on the floor. Put your left hand under your heat that will act as support. Place your right hand on your right side of the waist. Pull your knees together so that your legs are at a 45 degree formation. The resistance loop band should lie just above the knees. Now move your right knee so to spread your legs apart. The entire right leg should be stationary. Repeat for as long as you like. Also perform the same for the other leg.

Clamshell

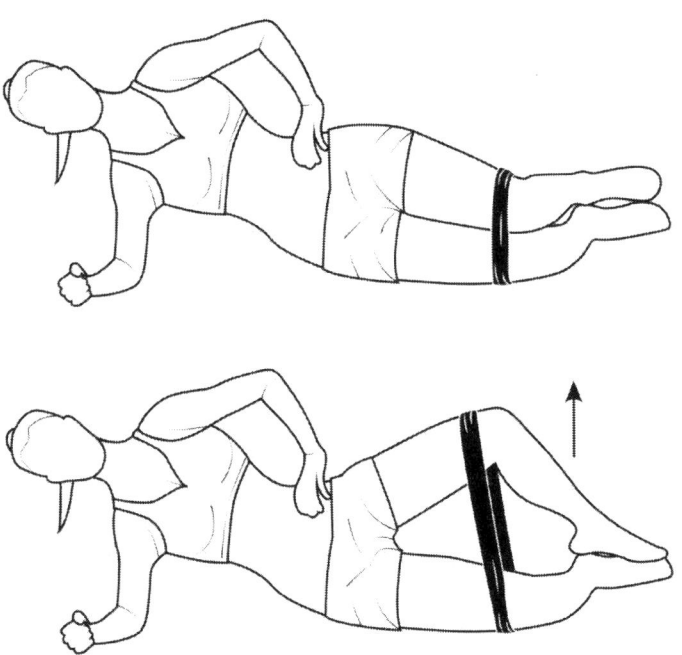

Lateral band walk. (Beginner)

To perform this exercise, simply wear the band in such a manner that it rests above your knees. The distance between your legs should be the distance between both of your shoulder. Now slightly bend your knees for about 20 degrees. Your entire spine should be inclined forward. Now move your right leg for about a foot to the right in such a way that the band exerts pressure on your hips. Now slowly bring in your other leg to the right side. Repeat the same procedure to the left side. You should alternate the right and the left for about 15 repetitions.

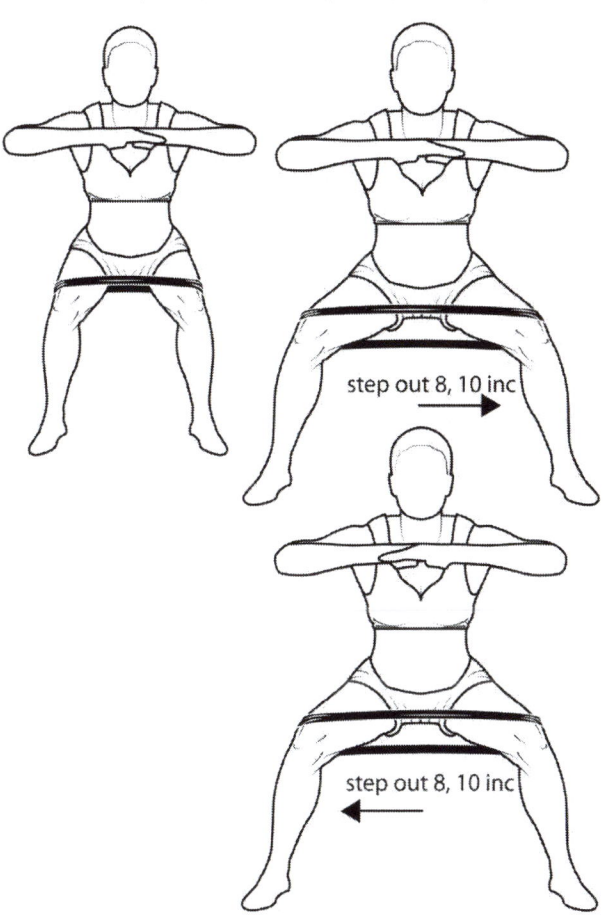

Squats. (Advance level)

Squat is one of the most effective forms of exercise that exists. It not only trains the lower body but also burns the fat at a rapid rate. The squat with the loop band is a bit different from the traditional form of squatting and it is difficult too. Place your knees around the band in a way that they rest just above your knees. Now slowly bring your upper body down while holding your hands together. Bring your body down until both of your hips are parallel to the ground. Repeat the exercise for 10 times in 3 sets.

Squats

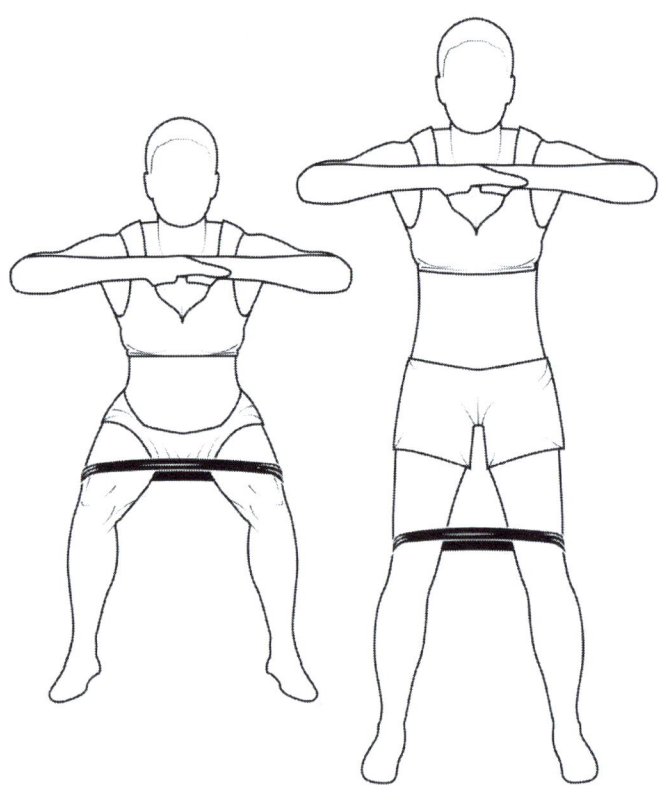

Leg extension. (Beginner)

The best exercise after squats for the lower body. It also trains multiple muscles with its movement. Sit on a chair and put the band in one of its legs so that it gets locked up. Put your right leg in the band and try to pull the band with an aim to make your leg parallel to the ground. This exercises affects your thigh majorly and your hips and calves in a minor way.

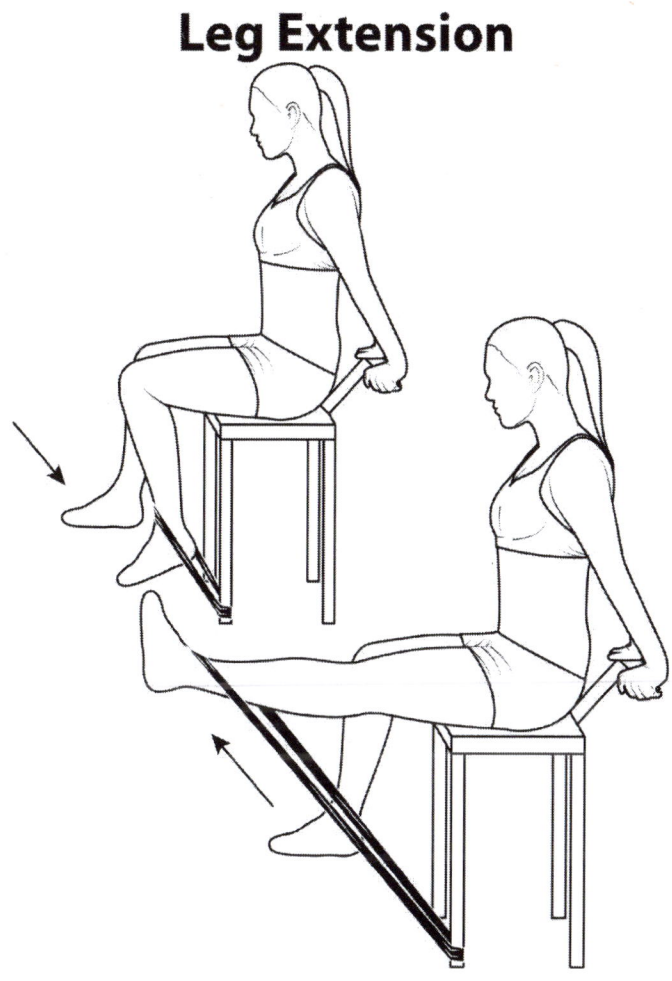

Hip thrust (Beginner)

Place both of your knees between the band so the band rests above your knee. Lie down on the floor in a relaxed manner. Raise your knees while the foot is still on the floor. The knee should point toward the sky. Now, while trying to pull your knees apart, raise your hip for about 7 to 10 inches above the ground. The more you stretch the band with your knees, the more your hip will rise above the ground. Repeat this exercise until you experience pain in your knees.

Hip Thrust

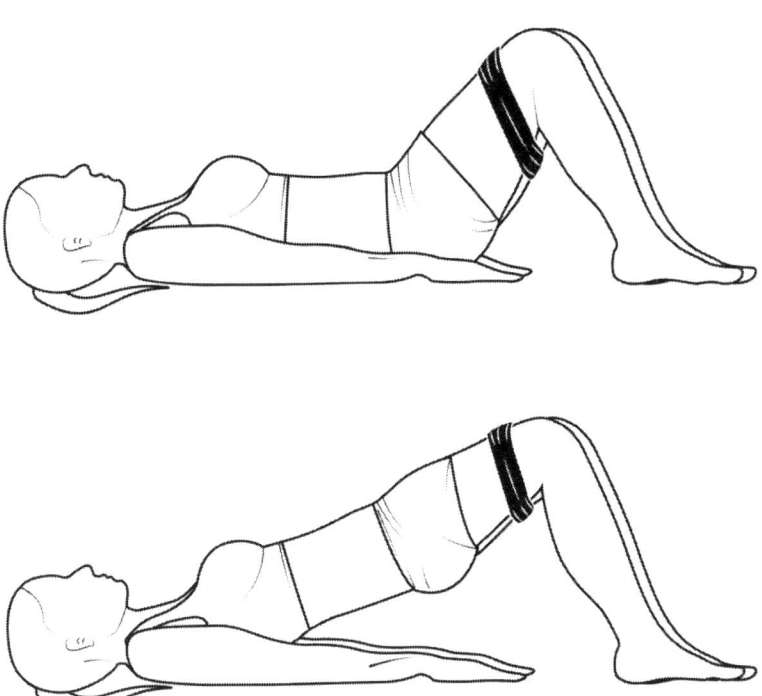

Bicycles (Advance level)

Even though the exercise is called the bicycles, the motion to perform the exercise is not circular but rather straight motion of your leg. Shoes are a must for this exercise. To perform this exercise, lie on the floor on your back. Place the resistance loop band around both of your foot so that it doesn't come loose. Now lie back with your hand behind your head. Slowly lift both of your feet in the air for about one foot. Now pull the right leg toward your stomach and at the same time try to touch the right knee with your left foot. Do the same for the left knee and right elbow. Repeat it for 6 to 10 time for 2 sets.

Bicycles

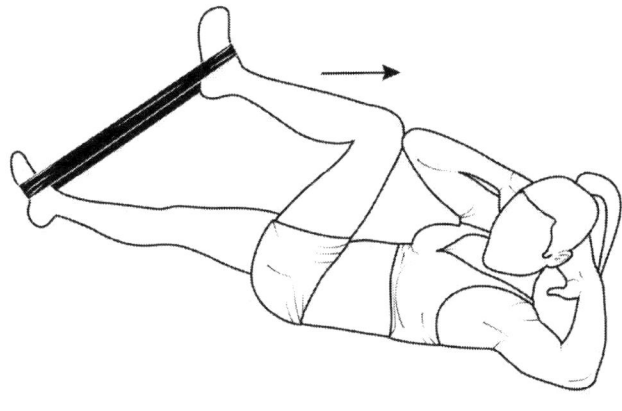

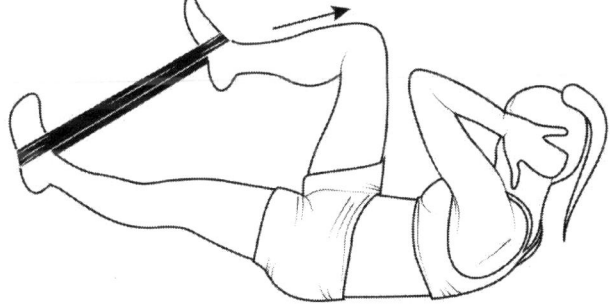

Glute trainer. (Beginner)

The purpose of this exercise is to train your glutes. To perform this exercise, stand on your legs. The distance between your feet should be about 6 inches and the resistance loop band should be suspended against your legs in the ankle region. Your hands should be on your waist in the respective side. Now bend your knee at a 45 degree angle so that the muscle is trained. The closer the loop band is to the ankle, the harder the exercise becomes. Now stay in this position for 5 sec and return to the initial position. Repeat the same with the left leg. Perform this routine for 20 times in 3 sets each.

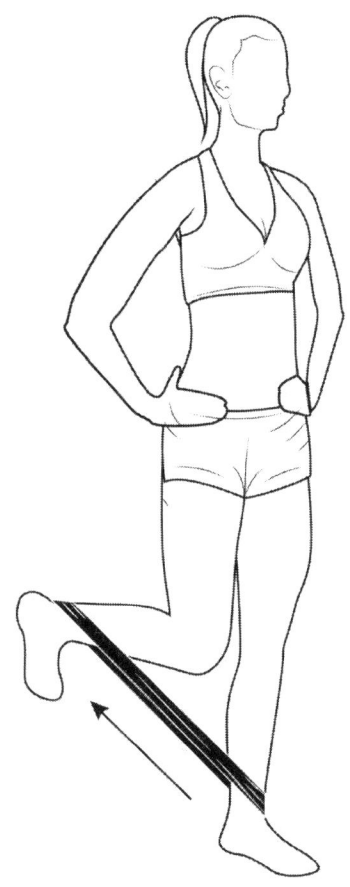

Glute Trainer

Abductor lift. (Advance level)

The abductor lift is an exercise to develop your hips in a way that the bystander will become instantly envious looking at your hips. These not only develop your hip but also fine tune them to near perfection level. To perform this exercise, lie down on the ground in a sideway manner by taking support with your hand. Put the resistance loop band around your leg. It should be at the region just above your ankle. Now try to pull your leg high up in the air. After the completion of the exercise, reverse your position and train your other leg. 12 repetitions for 3 sets.

Abductor Lift

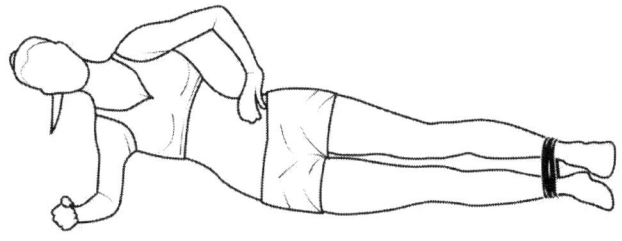

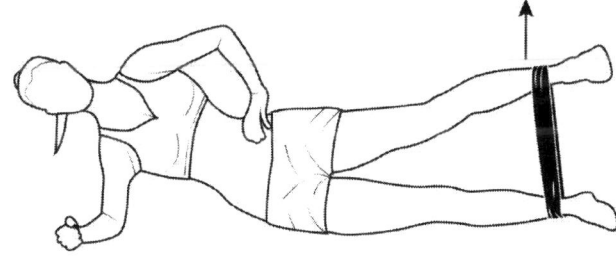

Chapter 7: Tips for using the resistance loop band and a word of caution.

I. Resistance loop band will increase your muscle strength only when you perform the full range of motion, in other case it will result in compound movement.

II. Resistance loop band should not be compared to free weights; they have their own advantages and disadvantages. It's best to utilize the full potential of the loop bands in its own unique way.

III. While performing an exercise, selection of the correct resistance loop band with adequate weight level is important for the exercise. Simple motion of the muscle will not develop it. Stress should be exerted on the muscle to make it very uncomfortable. More the stress, the more it develops.

IV. While performing an exercise, your mind should only be on the muscle targeted. Whether the muscle is moving correctly and experiencing pain. If not, then be sure that you are performing the exercise in a wrong manner.

V. If you don't feel any change, do not get discouraged, the resistance loop band method is a bit different. Your body will take some time to adapt and produce visible result

VI. If the results do not appear even after an elongated period of time, please consult a professional's help in this method of exercise to perform better.

VII. Do not perform the same exercise routine for a long period of time. Since the body adapts quickly, result will cease and the body doesn't improve. Add a little variety to your workout. Keep your body in the guessing state as to what will come next. This is the only method where your body will grow to the maximum.

On a final note, working out isn't an act to strengthen your body but an attempt to strengthen your life. A good and a healthy body lead to a healthy life. This resistance loop band is only an instrument in achieving this lifestyle. A lot of grip and determination is necessary to escape the traps of normal life to achieve the goals you want. Hope you find all the strengthen you need in an attempt to take charge of your life.

Alicia Labert

Printed in Great Britain
by Amazon